Pay Period: **Pay Date:**

Date	Starting Odometer	Starting Location	@ time	Ending Location	@ time	Route	Delays/ Detours
	Ending Odometer						
	Total Mileage						

reimbursement rate ¢/mile	fuel price $	costs to operate vehicle	tolls/fees	total hours	route notes
reimbursement total for today $	miles/gallon				

Date	Starting Odometer	Starting Location	@ time	Ending Location	@ time	Route	Delays/ Detours
	Ending Odometer						
	Total Mileage						

reimbursement rate ¢/mile	fuel price $	costs to operate vehicle	tolls/fees	total hours	route notes
reimbursement total for today $	miles/gallon				

Date	Starting Odometer	Starting Location	@ time	Ending Location	@ time	Route	Delays/ Detours
	Ending Odometer						
	Total Mileage						

reimbursement rate ¢/mile	fuel price $	costs to operate vehicle	tolls/fees	total hours	route notes
reimbursement total for today $	miles/gallon				

Pay Period: **Pay Date:**

Date	Starting Odometer	Starting Location	@ time	Ending Location	@ time	Route	Delays/Detours
	Ending Odometer						
	Total Mileage						

reimbursement rate	fuel price	costs to operate vehicle	tolls/fees	total hours	route notes
¢/mile	$				
reimbursement total for today $	miles/gallon				

Date	Starting Odometer	Starting Location	@ time	Ending Location	@ time	Route	Delays/Detours
	Ending Odometer						
	Total Mileage						

reimbursement rate	fuel price	costs to operate vehicle	tolls/fees	total hours	route notes
¢/mile	$				
reimbursement total for today $	miles/gallon				

Date	Starting Odometer	Starting Location	@ time	Ending Location	@ time	Route	Delays/Detours
	Ending Odometer						
	Total Mileage						

reimbursement rate	fuel price	costs to operate vehicle	tolls/fees	total hours	route notes
¢/mile	$				
reimbursement total for today $	miles/gallon				

Pay Period: **Pay Date:**

Date	Starting Odometer	Starting Location	@ time	Ending Location	@ time	Route	Delays/ Detours
	Ending Odometer						
	Total Mileage						
	reimbursement rate ¢/mile $	fuel price miles/gallon	costs to operate vehicle	tolls/fees	total hours	route notes	
	reimbursement total for today $						

Date	Starting Odometer	Starting Location	@ time	Ending Location	@ time	Route	Delays/ Detours
	Ending Odometer						
	Total Mileage						
	reimbursement rate ¢/mile $	fuel price miles/gallon	costs to operate vehicle	tolls/fees	total hours	route notes	
	reimbursement total for today $						

Date	Starting Odometer	Starting Location	@ time	Ending Location	@ time	Route	Delays/ Detours
	Ending Odometer						
	Total Mileage						
	reimbursement rate ¢/mile $	fuel price miles/gallon	costs to operate vehicle	tolls/fees	total hours	route notes	
	reimbursement total for today $						

Pay Period: **Pay Date:**

Date	Starting Odometer	Starting Location	@ time	Ending Location	@ time	Route	Delays/ Detours
	Ending Odometer						
	Total Mileage						

reimbursement rate	fuel price	costs to operate vehicle	tolls/fees	total hours	route notes
¢/mile $					
reimbursement total for today $	miles/gallon				

Date	Starting Odometer	Starting Location	@ time	Ending Location	@ time	Route	Delays/ Detours
	Ending Odometer						
	Total Mileage						

reimbursement rate	fuel price	costs to operate vehicle	tolls/fees	total hours	route notes
¢/mile $					
reimbursement total for today $	miles/gallon				

Date	Starting Odometer	Starting Location	@ time	Ending Location	@ time	Route	Delays/ Detours
	Ending Odometer						
	Total Mileage						

reimbursement rate	fuel price	costs to operate vehicle	tolls/fees	total hours	route notes
¢/mile $					
reimbursement total for today $	miles/gallon				

this pay period

date range _____   pay date _____

date worked	hours worked	hourly rate	x tax rate (= net)	+ mileage	= total net

totals

total miles driven _____
total fuel costs $
total expenses $

Pay Period: **Pay Date:**

Date	Starting Odometer	Starting Location	@ time	Ending Location	@ time	Route	Delays/ Detours
	Ending Odometer						
	Total Mileage						

reimbursement rate	fuel price	costs to operate vehicle	tolls/fees	total hours	route notes
¢/mile	$				
reimbursement total for today $	miles/gallon				

Date	Starting Odometer	Starting Location	@ time	Ending Location	@ time	Route	Delays/ Detours
	Ending Odometer						
	Total Mileage						

reimbursement rate	fuel price	costs to operate vehicle	tolls/fees	total hours	route notes
¢/mile	$				
reimbursement total for today $	miles/gallon				

Date	Starting Odometer	Starting Location	@ time	Ending Location	@ time	Route	Delays/ Detours
	Ending Odometer						
	Total Mileage						

reimbursement rate	fuel price	costs to operate vehicle	tolls/fees	total hours	route notes
¢/mile	$				
reimbursement total for today $	miles/gallon				

Pay Period: **Pay Date:**

Date	Starting Odometer	Starting Location	@ time	Ending Location	@ time	Route	Delays/Detours
	Ending Odometer						
	Total Mileage						

reimbursement rate ¢/mile	fuel price $	costs to operate vehicle	tolls/fees	total hours	route notes
reimbursement total for today $	miles/gallon				

Date	Starting Odometer	Starting Location	@ time	Ending Location	@ time	Route	Delays/Detours
	Ending Odometer						
	Total Mileage						

reimbursement rate ¢/mile	fuel price $	costs to operate vehicle	tolls/fees	total hours	route notes
reimbursement total for today $	miles/gallon				

Date	Starting Odometer	Starting Location	@ time	Ending Location	@ time	Route	Delays/Detours
	Ending Odometer						
	Total Mileage						

reimbursement rate ¢/mile	fuel price $	costs to operate vehicle	tolls/fees	total hours	route notes
reimbursement total for today $	miles/gallon				

Pay Period: **Pay Date:**

Date	Starting Odometer	Starting Location	@ time	Ending Location	@ time	Route	Delays/Detours
	Ending Odometer						
	Total Mileage						

reimbursement rate ¢/mile	fuel price $	costs to operate vehicle	tolls/fees	total hours	route notes
reimbursement total for today $	miles/gallon				

Date	Starting Odometer	Starting Location	@ time	Ending Location	@ time	Route	Delays/Detours
	Ending Odometer						
	Total Mileage						

reimbursement rate ¢/mile	fuel price $	costs to operate vehicle	tolls/fees	total hours	route notes
reimbursement total for today $	miles/gallon				

Date	Starting Odometer	Starting Location	@ time	Ending Location	@ time	Route	Delays/Detours
	Ending Odometer						
	Total Mileage						

reimbursement rate ¢/mile	fuel price $	costs to operate vehicle	tolls/fees	total hours	route notes
reimbursement total for today $	miles/gallon				

Pay Period: **Pay Date:**

Date	Starting Odometer	Starting Location	@ time	Ending Location	@ time	Route	Delays/Detours
	Ending Odometer						
	Total Mileage						
	reimbursement rate ¢/mile	fuel price $	costs to operate vehicle	tolls/fees	total hours	route notes	
	reimbursement total for today $	miles/gallon					

Date	Starting Odometer	Starting Location	@ time	Ending Location	@ time	Route	Delays/Detours
	Ending Odometer						
	Total Mileage						
	reimbursement rate ¢/mile	fuel price $	costs to operate vehicle	tolls/fees	total hours	route notes	
	reimbursement total for today $	miles/gallon					

Date	Starting Odometer	Starting Location	@ time	Ending Location	@ time	Route	Delays/Detours
	Ending Odometer						
	Total Mileage						
	reimbursement rate ¢/mile	fuel price $	costs to operate vehicle	tolls/fees	total hours	route notes	
	reimbursement total for today $	miles/gallon					

this pay period

date range _____   pay date _____

date worked	hours worked	hourly rate	× tax rate (= net)	+ mileage	= total net
totals					

total miles driven _____

total fuel costs $

total expenses $

Pay Period: **Pay Date:**

Date	Starting Odometer	Starting Location	@ time	Ending Location	@ time	Route	Delays/ Detours
	Ending Odometer						
	Total Mileage						
	reimbursement rate ¢/mile	fuel price $	costs to operate vehicle	tolls/fees	total hours	route notes	
	reimbursement total for today $	miles/gallon					

Date	Starting Odometer	Starting Location	@ time	Ending Location	@ time	Route	Delays/ Detours
	Ending Odometer						
	Total Mileage						
	reimbursement rate ¢/mile	fuel price $	costs to operate vehicle	tolls/fees	total hours	route notes	
	reimbursement total for today $	miles/gallon					

Date	Starting Odometer	Starting Location	@ time	Ending Location	@ time	Route	Delays/ Detours
	Ending Odometer						
	Total Mileage						
	reimbursement rate ¢/mile	fuel price $	costs to operate vehicle	tolls/fees	total hours	route notes	
	reimbursement total for today $	miles/gallon					

Pay Period: **Pay Date:**

Date	Starting Odometer	Starting Location	@ time	Ending Location	@ time	Route	Delays/Detours
	Ending Odometer						
	Total Mileage						
	reimbursement rate ¢/mile	fuel price $	costs to operate vehicle	tolls/fees	total hours	route notes	
	reimbursement total for today $	miles/gallon					

Date	Starting Odometer	Starting Location	@ time	Ending Location	@ time	Route	Delays/Detours
	Ending Odometer						
	Total Mileage						
	reimbursement rate ¢/mile	fuel price $	costs to operate vehicle	tolls/fees	total hours	route notes	
	reimbursement total for today $	miles/gallon					

Date	Starting Odometer	Starting Location	@ time	Ending Location	@ time	Route	Delays/Detours
	Ending Odometer						
	Total Mileage						
	reimbursement rate ¢/mile	fuel price $	costs to operate vehicle	tolls/fees	total hours	route notes	
	reimbursement total for today $	miles/gallon					

Pay Period: **Pay Date:**

Date	Starting Odometer	Starting Location	@ time	Ending Location	@ time	Route	Delays/ Detours
	Ending Odometer						
	Total Mileage						

reimbursement rate ¢/mile	fuel price $	costs to operate vehicle	tolls/fees	total hours	route notes
reimbursement total for today $	miles/gallon				

Date	Starting Odometer	Starting Location	@ time	Ending Location	@ time	Route	Delays/ Detours
	Ending Odometer						
	Total Mileage						

reimbursement rate ¢/mile	fuel price $	costs to operate vehicle	tolls/fees	total hours	route notes
reimbursement total for today $	miles/gallon				

Date	Starting Odometer	Starting Location	@ time	Ending Location	@ time	Route	Delays/ Detours
	Ending Odometer						
	Total Mileage						

reimbursement rate ¢/mile	fuel price $	costs to operate vehicle	tolls/fees	total hours	route notes
reimbursement total for today $	miles/gallon				

Pay Period: **Pay Date:**

Date	Starting Odometer	Starting Location	@ time	Ending Location	@ time	Route	Delays/Detours
	Ending Odometer						
	Total Mileage						

reimbursement rate ¢/mile	fuel price $	costs to operate vehicle	tolls/fees	total hours	route notes
reimbursement total for today $	miles/gallon				

Date	Starting Odometer	Starting Location	@ time	Ending Location	@ time	Route	Delays/Detours
	Ending Odometer						
	Total Mileage						

reimbursement rate ¢/mile	fuel price $	costs to operate vehicle	tolls/fees	total hours	route notes
reimbursement total for today $	miles/gallon				

Date	Starting Odometer	Starting Location	@ time	Ending Location	@ time	Route	Delays/Detours
	Ending Odometer						
	Total Mileage						

reimbursement rate ¢/mile	fuel price $	costs to operate vehicle	tolls/fees	total hours	route notes
reimbursement total for today $	miles/gallon				

this pay period

date range _____   pay date _____

date worked	hours worked	hourly rate	x tax rate (= net)	+ mileage	= total net
totals					

total miles driven _____

total fuel costs $

total expenses $

Pay Period: **Pay Date:**

Date	Starting Odometer	Starting Location	@ time	Ending Location	@ time	Route	Delays/Detours
	Ending Odometer						
	Total Mileage						

reimbursement rate	fuel price	costs to operate vehicle	tolls/fees	total hours	route notes
¢/mile $	miles/gallon			☐	
reimbursement total for today $					

Date	Starting Odometer	Starting Location	@ time	Ending Location	@ time	Route	Delays/Detours
	Ending Odometer						
	Total Mileage						

reimbursement rate	fuel price	costs to operate vehicle	tolls/fees	total hours	route notes
¢/mile $	miles/gallon			☐	
reimbursement total for today $					

Date	Starting Odometer	Starting Location	@ time	Ending Location	@ time	Route	Delays/Detours
	Ending Odometer						
	Total Mileage						

reimbursement rate	fuel price	costs to operate vehicle	tolls/fees	total hours	route notes
¢/mile $	miles/gallon			☐	
reimbursement total for today $					

Pay Period: **Pay Date:**

Date	Starting Odometer	Starting Location	@ time	Ending Location	@ time	Route	Delays/ Detours
	Ending Odometer						
	Total Mileage						
	reimbursement rate ¢/mile	fuel price $	costs to operate vehicle	tolls/fees	total hours	route notes	
	reimbursement total for today $	miles/gallon					

Date	Starting Odometer	Starting Location	@ time	Ending Location	@ time	Route	Delays/ Detours
	Ending Odometer						
	Total Mileage						
	reimbursement rate ¢/mile	fuel price $	costs to operate vehicle	tolls/fees	total hours	route notes	
	reimbursement total for today $	miles/gallon					

Date	Starting Odometer	Starting Location	@ time	Ending Location	@ time	Route	Delays/ Detours
	Ending Odometer						
	Total Mileage						
	reimbursement rate ¢/mile	fuel price $	costs to operate vehicle	tolls/fees	total hours	route notes	
	reimbursement total for today $	miles/gallon					

Pay Period:　　　　　　　　　　　　　　　　**Pay Date:**

Date	Starting Odometer	Starting Location	@ time	Ending Location	@ time	Route	Delays/Detours
	Ending Odometer						
	Total Mileage						

reimbursement rate ¢/mile	fuel price $	costs to operate vehicle	tolls/fees	total hours	route notes
reimbursement total for today $	miles/gallon				

Date	Starting Odometer	Starting Location	@ time	Ending Location	@ time	Route	Delays/Detours
	Ending Odometer						
	Total Mileage						

reimbursement rate ¢/mile	fuel price $	costs to operate vehicle	tolls/fees	total hours	route notes
reimbursement total for today $	miles/gallon				

Date	Starting Odometer	Starting Location	@ time	Ending Location	@ time	Route	Delays/Detours
	Ending Odometer						
	Total Mileage						

reimbursement rate ¢/mile	fuel price $	costs to operate vehicle	tolls/fees	total hours	route notes
reimbursement total for today $	miles/gallon				

Pay Period: **Pay Date:**

Entry 1

Date	Starting Odometer	Starting Location	@ time	Ending Location	@ time	Route	Delays/ Detours
	Ending Odometer						
	Total Mileage						

reimbursement rate ¢/mile	fuel price $	costs to operate vehicle	tolls/fees	total hours	route notes
reimbursement total for today $	miles/gallon				

Entry 2

Date	Starting Odometer	Starting Location	@ time	Ending Location	@ time	Route	Delays/ Detours
	Ending Odometer						
	Total Mileage						

reimbursement rate ¢/mile	fuel price $	costs to operate vehicle	tolls/fees	total hours	route notes
reimbursement total for today $	miles/gallon				

Entry 3

Date	Starting Odometer	Starting Location	@ time	Ending Location	@ time	Route	Delays/ Detours
	Ending Odometer						
	Total Mileage						

reimbursement rate ¢/mile	fuel price $	costs to operate vehicle	tolls/fees	total hours	route notes
reimbursement total for today $	miles/gallon				

this pay period

date range _____ pay date _____

date worked	hours worked	hourly rate	x tax rate (= net)	+ mileage	= total net

totals

total miles driven _____
total fuel costs $
total expenses $

Pay Period: **Pay Date:**

Date	Starting Odometer	Starting Location	@ time	Ending Location	@ time	Route	Delays/Detours
	Ending Odometer						
	Total Mileage						

reimbursement rate ¢/mile	fuel price $	costs to operate vehicle	tolls/fees	total hours	route notes
reimbursement total for today $	miles/gallon				

Date	Starting Odometer	Starting Location	@ time	Ending Location	@ time	Route	Delays/Detours
	Ending Odometer						
	Total Mileage						

reimbursement rate ¢/mile	fuel price $	costs to operate vehicle	tolls/fees	total hours	route notes
reimbursement total for today $	miles/gallon				

Date	Starting Odometer	Starting Location	@ time	Ending Location	@ time	Route	Delays/Detours
	Ending Odometer						
	Total Mileage						

reimbursement rate ¢/mile	fuel price $	costs to operate vehicle	tolls/fees	total hours	route notes
reimbursement total for today $	miles/gallon				

Pay Period:　　　　　　　　　　　　　　　　**Pay Date:**

Date	Starting Odometer	Starting Location	@ time	Ending Location	@ time	Route	Delays/Detours
	Ending Odometer						
	Total Mileage						

reimbursement rate ¢/mile	fuel price $	costs to operate vehicle	tolls/fees	total hours	route notes
reimbursement total for today $	miles/gallon				

Date	Starting Odometer	Starting Location	@ time	Ending Location	@ time	Route	Delays/Detours
	Ending Odometer						
	Total Mileage						

reimbursement rate ¢/mile	fuel price $	costs to operate vehicle	tolls/fees	total hours	route notes
reimbursement total for today $	miles/gallon				

Date	Starting Odometer	Starting Location	@ time	Ending Location	@ time	Route	Delays/Detours
	Ending Odometer						
	Total Mileage						

reimbursement rate ¢/mile	fuel price $	costs to operate vehicle	tolls/fees	total hours	route notes
reimbursement total for today $	miles/gallon				

Pay Period: **Pay Date:**

Date	Starting Odometer	Starting Location	@ time	Ending Location	@ time	Route	Delays/Detours
○	Ending Odometer						
	Total Mileage						

reimbursement rate ¢/mile	fuel price $	costs to operate vehicle	tolls/fees	total hours	route notes
reimbursement total for today $	miles/gallon				

Date	Starting Odometer	Starting Location	@ time	Ending Location	@ time	Route	Delays/Detours
○	Ending Odometer						
	Total Mileage						

reimbursement rate ¢/mile	fuel price $	costs to operate vehicle	tolls/fees	total hours	route notes
reimbursement total for today $	miles/gallon				

Date	Starting Odometer	Starting Location	@ time	Ending Location	@ time	Route	Delays/Detours
○	Ending Odometer						
	Total Mileage						

reimbursement rate ¢/mile	fuel price $	costs to operate vehicle	tolls/fees	total hours	route notes
reimbursement total for today $	miles/gallon				

Pay Period: **Pay Date:**

Date	Starting Odometer	Starting Location	@ time	Ending Location	@ time	Route	Delays/Detours
	Ending Odometer						
	Total Mileage						

reimbursement rate ¢/mile	fuel price $	costs to operate vehicle	tolls/fees	total hours	route notes
reimbursement total for today $	miles/gallon				

Date	Starting Odometer	Starting Location	@ time	Ending Location	@ time	Route	Delays/Detours
	Ending Odometer						
	Total Mileage						

reimbursement rate ¢/mile	fuel price $	costs to operate vehicle	tolls/fees	total hours	route notes
reimbursement total for today $	miles/gallon				

Date	Starting Odometer	Starting Location	@ time	Ending Location	@ time	Route	Delays/Detours
	Ending Odometer						
	Total Mileage						

reimbursement rate ¢/mile	fuel price $	costs to operate vehicle	tolls/fees	total hours	route notes
reimbursement total for today $	miles/gallon				

this pay period

date range _____ pay date _____

date worked	hours worked	hourly rate	x tax rate (= net)	+ mileage	= total net
totals					

total miles driven _____

total fuel costs $

total expenses $

Pay Period: **Pay Date:**

Date	Starting Odometer	Starting Location	@ time	Ending Location	@ time	Route	Delays/Detours
	Ending Odometer						
	Total Mileage						

reimbursement rate ¢/mile	fuel price $	costs to operate vehicle	tolls/fees	total hours	route notes
reimbursement total for today $	miles/gallon				

Date	Starting Odometer	Starting Location	@ time	Ending Location	@ time	Route	Delays/Detours
	Ending Odometer						
	Total Mileage						

reimbursement rate ¢/mile	fuel price $	costs to operate vehicle	tolls/fees	total hours	route notes
reimbursement total for today $	miles/gallon				

Date	Starting Odometer	Starting Location	@ time	Ending Location	@ time	Route	Delays/Detours
	Ending Odometer						
	Total Mileage						

reimbursement rate ¢/mile	fuel price $	costs to operate vehicle	tolls/fees	total hours	route notes
reimbursement total for today $	miles/gallon				

Pay Period: **Pay Date:**

Date	Starting Odometer	Starting Location	@ time	Ending Location	@ time	Route	Delays/ Detours
	Ending Odometer						
	Total Mileage						
	reimbursement rate ¢/mile	fuel price $	costs to operate vehicle	tolls/fees	total hours	route notes	
	reimbursement total for today $	miles/gallon					

Date	Starting Odometer	Starting Location	@ time	Ending Location	@ time	Route	Delays/ Detours
	Ending Odometer						
	Total Mileage						
	reimbursement rate ¢/mile	fuel price $	costs to operate vehicle	tolls/fees	total hours	route notes	
	reimbursement total for today $	miles/gallon					

Date	Starting Odometer	Starting Location	@ time	Ending Location	@ time	Route	Delays/ Detours
	Ending Odometer						
	Total Mileage						
	reimbursement rate ¢/mile	fuel price $	costs to operate vehicle	tolls/fees	total hours	route notes	
	reimbursement total for today $	miles/gallon					

Pay Period: **Pay Date:**

Date	Starting Odometer	Starting Location	@ time	Ending Location	@ time	Route	Delays/Detours
	Ending Odometer						
	Total Mileage						

reimbursement rate ¢/mile	fuel price $	costs to operate vehicle	tolls/fees	total hours	route notes
reimbursement total for today $	miles/gallon				

Date	Starting Odometer	Starting Location	@ time	Ending Location	@ time	Route	Delays/Detours
	Ending Odometer						
	Total Mileage						

reimbursement rate ¢/mile	fuel price $	costs to operate vehicle	tolls/fees	total hours	route notes
reimbursement total for today $	miles/gallon				

Date	Starting Odometer	Starting Location	@ time	Ending Location	@ time	Route	Delays/Detours
	Ending Odometer						
	Total Mileage						

reimbursement rate ¢/mile	fuel price $	costs to operate vehicle	tolls/fees	total hours	route notes
reimbursement total for today $	miles/gallon				

Pay Period: **Pay Date:**

Date	Starting Odometer	Starting Location	@ time	Ending Location	@ time	Route	Delays/ Detours
	Ending Odometer						
	Total Mileage						
reimbursement rate ¢/mile	fuel price $	costs to operate vehicle	tolls/fees	total hours	route notes		
reimbursement total for today $	miles/gallon						

Date	Starting Odometer	Starting Location	@ time	Ending Location	@ time	Route	Delays/ Detours
	Ending Odometer						
	Total Mileage						
reimbursement rate ¢/mile	fuel price $	costs to operate vehicle	tolls/fees	total hours	route notes		
reimbursement total for today $	miles/gallon						

Date	Starting Odometer	Starting Location	@ time	Ending Location	@ time	Route	Delays/ Detours
	Ending Odometer						
	Total Mileage						
reimbursement rate ¢/mile	fuel price $	costs to operate vehicle	tolls/fees	total hours	route notes		
reimbursement total for today $	miles/gallon						

this pay period

date range _____   pay date _____

date worked	hours worked	hourly rate	× tax rate (= net)	+ mileage	= total net

totals

total miles driven _____
total fuel costs $
total expenses $

Pay Period: . **Pay Date:**

Date	Starting Odometer / Ending Odometer / Total Mileage	Starting Location	@ time	Ending Location	@ time	Route	Delays/ Detours
○							

reimbursement rate ¢/mile   fuel price $ costs to operate vehicle   tolls/fees   total hours □   route notes

reimbursement total for today $ miles/gallon

Date	Starting Odometer / Ending Odometer / Total Mileage	Starting Location	@ time	Ending Location	@ time	Route	Delays/ Detours
○							

reimbursement rate ¢/mile   fuel price $ costs to operate vehicle   tolls/fees   total hours □   route notes

reimbursement total for today $ miles/gallon

Date	Starting Odometer / Ending Odometer / Total Mileage	Starting Location	@ time	Ending Location	@ time	Route	Delays/ Detours
○							

reimbursement rate ¢/mile   fuel price $ costs to operate vehicle   tolls/fees   total hours □   route notes

reimbursement total for today $ miles/gallon

Pay Period: **Pay Date:**

Date	Starting Odometer	Starting Location	@ time	Ending Location	@ time	Route	Delays/ Detours
○							
	Ending Odometer						
	Total Mileage						

reimbursement rate ¢/mile	fuel price $	costs to operate vehicle	tolls/fees	total hours	route notes
reimbursement total for today $	miles/gallon				

Date	Starting Odometer	Starting Location	@ time	Ending Location	@ time	Route	Delays/ Detours
○							
	Ending Odometer						
	Total Mileage						

reimbursement rate ¢/mile	fuel price $	costs to operate vehicle	tolls/fees	total hours	route notes
reimbursement total for today $	miles/gallon				

Date	Starting Odometer	Starting Location	@ time	Ending Location	@ time	Route	Delays/ Detours
○							
	Ending Odometer						
	Total Mileage						

reimbursement rate ¢/mile	fuel price $	costs to operate vehicle	tolls/fees	total hours	route notes
reimbursement total for today $	miles/gallon				

Pay Period: **Pay Date:**

Date	Starting Odometer	Starting Location	@ time	Ending Location	@ time	Route	Delays/Detours
	Ending Odometer						
	Total Mileage						

reimbursement rate ¢/mile	fuel price $	costs to operate vehicle	tolls/fees	total hours	route notes
reimbursement total for today $	miles/gallon				

Date	Starting Odometer	Starting Location	@ time	Ending Location	@ time	Route	Delays/Detours
	Ending Odometer						
	Total Mileage						

reimbursement rate ¢/mile	fuel price $	costs to operate vehicle	tolls/fees	total hours	route notes
reimbursement total for today $	miles/gallon				

Date	Starting Odometer	Starting Location	@ time	Ending Location	@ time	Route	Delays/Detours
	Ending Odometer						
	Total Mileage						

reimbursement rate ¢/mile	fuel price $	costs to operate vehicle	tolls/fees	total hours	route notes
reimbursement total for today $	miles/gallon				

Pay Period: **Pay Date:**

Date	Starting Odometer	Starting Location	@ time	Ending Location	@ time	Route	Delays/Detours
	Ending Odometer						
	Total Mileage						

reimbursement rate ¢/mile	fuel price $	costs to operate vehicle	tolls/fees	total hours	route notes
reimbursement total for today $	miles/gallon				

Date	Starting Odometer	Starting Location	@ time	Ending Location	@ time	Route	Delays/Detours
	Ending Odometer						
	Total Mileage						

reimbursement rate ¢/mile	fuel price $	costs to operate vehicle	tolls/fees	total hours	route notes
reimbursement total for today $	miles/gallon				

Date	Starting Odometer	Starting Location	@ time	Ending Location	@ time	Route	Delays/Detours
	Ending Odometer						
	Total Mileage						

reimbursement rate ¢/mile	fuel price $	costs to operate vehicle	tolls/fees	total hours	route notes
reimbursement total for today $	miles/gallon				

this pay period

date range _____   pay date _____

date worked	hours worked	hourly rate	x tax rate (= net)	+ mileage	= total net

totals

total miles driven _____
total fuel costs $
total expenses $

Pay Period:　　　　　　　　　　　　　　　　　**Pay Date:**

Date	Starting Odometer	Starting Location	@ time	Ending Location	@ time	Route	Delays/ Detours
	Ending Odometer						
	Total Mileage						

reimbursement rate ¢/mile	fuel price $	costs to operate vehicle	tolls/fees	total hours	route notes
reimbursement total for today $	miles/gallon				

Date	Starting Odometer	Starting Location	@ time	Ending Location	@ time	Route	Delays/ Detours
	Ending Odometer						
	Total Mileage						

reimbursement rate ¢/mile	fuel price $	costs to operate vehicle	tolls/fees	total hours	route notes
reimbursement total for today $	miles/gallon				

Date	Starting Odometer	Starting Location	@ time	Ending Location	@ time	Route	Delays/ Detours
	Ending Odometer						
	Total Mileage						

reimbursement rate ¢/mile	fuel price $	costs to operate vehicle	tolls/fees	total hours	route notes
reimbursement total for today $	miles/gallon				

Pay Period: **Pay Date:**

Entry 1

Date	Starting Odometer	Starting Location	@ time	Ending Location	@ time	Route	Delays/Detours
	Ending Odometer						
	Total Mileage						

reimbursement rate ¢/mile	fuel price $	costs to operate vehicle	tolls/fees	total hours	route notes
reimbursement total for today $	miles/gallon				

Entry 2

Date	Starting Odometer	Starting Location	@ time	Ending Location	@ time	Route	Delays/Detours
	Ending Odometer						
	Total Mileage						

reimbursement rate ¢/mile	fuel price $	costs to operate vehicle	tolls/fees	total hours	route notes
reimbursement total for today $	miles/gallon				

Entry 3

Date	Starting Odometer	Starting Location	@ time	Ending Location	@ time	Route	Delays/Detours
	Ending Odometer						
	Total Mileage						

reimbursement rate ¢/mile	fuel price $	costs to operate vehicle	tolls/fees	total hours	route notes
reimbursement total for today $	miles/gallon				

Pay Period: **Pay Date:**

Date	Starting Odometer	Starting Location	@ time	Ending Location	@ time	Route	Delays/ Detours
	Ending Odometer						
	Total Mileage						

reimbursement rate ¢/mile	fuel price $	costs to operate vehicle	tolls/fees	total hours	route notes
reimbursement total for today $	miles/gallon				

Date	Starting Odometer	Starting Location	@ time	Ending Location	@ time	Route	Delays/ Detours
	Ending Odometer						
	Total Mileage						

reimbursement rate ¢/mile	fuel price $	costs to operate vehicle	tolls/fees	total hours	route notes
reimbursement total for today $	miles/gallon				

Date	Starting Odometer	Starting Location	@ time	Ending Location	@ time	Route	Delays/ Detours
	Ending Odometer						
	Total Mileage						

reimbursement rate ¢/mile	fuel price $	costs to operate vehicle	tolls/fees	total hours	route notes
reimbursement total for today $	miles/gallon				

Pay Period: **Pay Date:**

Date	Starting Odometer	Starting Location	@ time	Ending Location	@ time	Route	Delays/Detours
	Ending Odometer						
	Total Mileage						

reimbursement rate ¢/mile	fuel price $	costs to operate vehicle	tolls/fees	total hours	route notes
reimbursement total for today $	miles/gallon				

Date	Starting Odometer	Starting Location	@ time	Ending Location	@ time	Route	Delays/Detours
	Ending Odometer						
	Total Mileage						

reimbursement rate ¢/mile	fuel price $	costs to operate vehicle	tolls/fees	total hours	route notes
reimbursement total for today $	miles/gallon				

Date	Starting Odometer	Starting Location	@ time	Ending Location	@ time	Route	Delays/Detours
	Ending Odometer						
	Total Mileage						

reimbursement rate ¢/mile	fuel price $	costs to operate vehicle	tolls/fees	total hours	route notes
reimbursement total for today $	miles/gallon				

this pay period

date range _____   pay date _____

date worked	hours worked	hourly rate	× tax rate (= net)	+ mileage	= total net
totals					

total miles driven _____
total fuel costs $
total expenses $

Pay Period: **Pay Date:**

Date	Starting Odometer	Starting Location	@ time	Ending Location	@ time	Route	Delays/Detours
	Ending Odometer						
	Total Mileage						

| reimbursement rate ¢/mile | fuel price $ miles/gallon | costs to operate vehicle | tolls/fees | total hours | route notes | | |
| reimbursement total for today $ | | | | | | | |

Date	Starting Odometer	Starting Location	@ time	Ending Location	@ time	Route	Delays/Detours
	Ending Odometer						
	Total Mileage						

| reimbursement rate ¢/mile | fuel price $ miles/gallon | costs to operate vehicle | tolls/fees | total hours | route notes | | |
| reimbursement total for today $ | | | | | | | |

Date	Starting Odometer	Starting Location	@ time	Ending Location	@ time	Route	Delays/Detours
	Ending Odometer						
	Total Mileage						

| reimbursement rate ¢/mile | fuel price $ miles/gallon | costs to operate vehicle | tolls/fees | total hours | route notes | | |
| reimbursement total for today $ | | | | | | | |

Pay Period: **Pay Date:**

Date	Starting Odometer	Starting Location	@ time	Ending Location	@ time	Route	Delays/Detours
	Ending Odometer						
	Total Mileage						

reimbursement rate ¢/mile	fuel price $	costs to operate vehicle	tolls/fees	total hours	route notes
reimbursement total for today $	miles/gallon				

Date	Starting Odometer	Starting Location	@ time	Ending Location	@ time	Route	Delays/Detours
	Ending Odometer						
	Total Mileage						

reimbursement rate ¢/mile	fuel price $	costs to operate vehicle	tolls/fees	total hours	route notes
reimbursement total for today $	miles/gallon				

Date	Starting Odometer	Starting Location	@ time	Ending Location	@ time	Route	Delays/Detours
	Ending Odometer						
	Total Mileage						

reimbursement rate ¢/mile	fuel price $	costs to operate vehicle	tolls/fees	total hours	route notes
reimbursement total for today $	miles/gallon				

Pay Period: **Pay Date:**

Date	Starting Odometer	Starting Location	@ time	Ending Location	@ time	Route	Delays/Detours
	Ending Odometer						
	Total Mileage						

reimbursement rate ¢/mile	fuel price $	costs to operate vehicle	tolls/fees	total hours	route notes
reimbursement total for today $	miles/gallon				

Date	Starting Odometer	Starting Location	@ time	Ending Location	@ time	Route	Delays/Detours
	Ending Odometer						
	Total Mileage						

reimbursement rate ¢/mile	fuel price $	costs to operate vehicle	tolls/fees	total hours	route notes
reimbursement total for today $	miles/gallon				

Date	Starting Odometer	Starting Location	@ time	Ending Location	@ time	Route	Delays/Detours
	Ending Odometer						
	Total Mileage						

reimbursement rate ¢/mile	fuel price $	costs to operate vehicle	tolls/fees	total hours	route notes
reimbursement total for today $	miles/gallon				

Pay Period: **Pay Date:**

Entry 1

Date	Starting Odometer	Starting Location	@ time	Ending Location	@ time	Route	Delays/Detours
○							
	Ending Odometer						
	Total Mileage						

reimbursement rate ¢/mile	fuel price $	costs to operate vehicle	tolls/fees	total hours	route notes
reimbursement total for today $	miles/gallon				

Entry 2

Date	Starting Odometer	Starting Location	@ time	Ending Location	@ time	Route	Delays/Detours
○							
	Ending Odometer						
	Total Mileage						

reimbursement rate ¢/mile	fuel price $	costs to operate vehicle	tolls/fees	total hours	route notes
reimbursement total for today $	miles/gallon				

Entry 3

Date	Starting Odometer	Starting Location	@ time	Ending Location	@ time	Route	Delays/Detours
○							
	Ending Odometer						
	Total Mileage						

reimbursement rate ¢/mile	fuel price $	costs to operate vehicle	tolls/fees	total hours	route notes
reimbursement total for today $	miles/gallon				

this pay period

date range _____   pay date _____

date worked	hours worked	hourly rate	× tax rate (= net)	+ mileage	= total net

totals

total miles driven _____
total fuel costs $
total expenses $

Pay Period: **Pay Date:**

Date	Starting Odometer	Starting Location	@ time	Ending Location	@ time	Route	Delays/Detours
	Ending Odometer						
	Total Mileage						

reimbursement rate	fuel price	costs to operate vehicle	tolls/fees	total hours	route notes
¢/mile	$				
reimbursement total for today	miles/gallon				
$					

Date	Starting Odometer	Starting Location	@ time	Ending Location	@ time	Route	Delays/Detours
	Ending Odometer						
	Total Mileage						

reimbursement rate	fuel price	costs to operate vehicle	tolls/fees	total hours	route notes
¢/mile	$				
reimbursement total for today	miles/gallon				
$					

Date	Starting Odometer	Starting Location	@ time	Ending Location	@ time	Route	Delays/Detours
	Ending Odometer						
	Total Mileage						

reimbursement rate	fuel price	costs to operate vehicle	tolls/fees	total hours	route notes
¢/mile	$				
reimbursement total for today	miles/gallon				
$					

Pay Period: **Pay Date:**

Date	Starting Odometer	Starting Location	@ time	Ending Location	@ time	Route	Delays/Detours
	Ending Odometer						
	Total Mileage						
	reimbursement rate ¢/mile	fuel price $	costs to operate vehicle	tolls/fees	total hours	route notes	
	reimbursement total for today $	miles/gallon					

Date	Starting Odometer	Starting Location	@ time	Ending Location	@ time	Route	Delays/Detours
	Ending Odometer						
	Total Mileage						
	reimbursement rate ¢/mile	fuel price $	costs to operate vehicle	tolls/fees	total hours	route notes	
	reimbursement total for today $	miles/gallon					

Date	Starting Odometer	Starting Location	@ time	Ending Location	@ time	Route	Delays/Detours
	Ending Odometer						
	Total Mileage						
	reimbursement rate ¢/mile	fuel price $	costs to operate vehicle	tolls/fees	total hours	route notes	
	reimbursement total for today $	miles/gallon					

Pay Period: **Pay Date:**

Date	Starting Odometer	Starting Location	@ time	Ending Location	@ time	Route	Delays/ Detours
	Ending Odometer						
	Total Mileage						

reimbursement rate ¢/mile	fuel price $	costs to operate vehicle	tolls/fees	total hours	route notes
reimbursement total for today $	miles/gallon				

Date	Starting Odometer	Starting Location	@ time	Ending Location	@ time	Route	Delays/ Detours
	Ending Odometer						
	Total Mileage						

reimbursement rate ¢/mile	fuel price $	costs to operate vehicle	tolls/fees	total hours	route notes
reimbursement total for today $	miles/gallon				

Date	Starting Odometer	Starting Location	@ time	Ending Location	@ time	Route	Delays/ Detours
	Ending Odometer						
	Total Mileage						

reimbursement rate ¢/mile	fuel price $	costs to operate vehicle	tolls/fees	total hours	route notes
reimbursement total for today $	miles/gallon				

Pay Period: **Pay Date:**

Date	Starting Odometer	Starting Location	@ time	Ending Location	@ time	Route	Delays/ Detours
	Ending Odometer						
	Total Mileage						

reimbursement rate ¢/mile	fuel price $	costs to operate vehicle	tolls/fees	total hours	route notes
reimbursement total for today $	miles/gallon				

Date	Starting Odometer	Starting Location	@ time	Ending Location	@ time	Route	Delays/ Detours
	Ending Odometer						
	Total Mileage						

reimbursement rate ¢/mile	fuel price $	costs to operate vehicle	tolls/fees	total hours	route notes
reimbursement total for today $	miles/gallon				

Date	Starting Odometer	Starting Location	@ time	Ending Location	@ time	Route	Delays/ Detours
	Ending Odometer						
	Total Mileage						

reimbursement rate ¢/mile	fuel price $	costs to operate vehicle	tolls/fees	total hours	route notes
reimbursement total for today $	miles/gallon				

this pay period

date range _____   pay date _____

			×		
date worked	hours worked	hourly rate	tax rate (= net)	+ mileage	= total net

totals

total miles driven _____

total fuel costs $

total expenses $

Pay Period: **Pay Date:**

Date	Starting Odometer	Starting Location	@ time	Ending Location	@ time	Route	Delays/ Detours
	Ending Odometer						
	Total Mileage						

reimbursement rate ¢/mile	fuel price $	costs to operate vehicle	tolls/fees	total hours	route notes
reimbursement total for today $	miles/gallon				

Date	Starting Odometer	Starting Location	@ time	Ending Location	@ time	Route	Delays/ Detours
	Ending Odometer						
	Total Mileage						

reimbursement rate ¢/mile	fuel price $	costs to operate vehicle	tolls/fees	total hours	route notes
reimbursement total for today $	miles/gallon				

Date	Starting Odometer	Starting Location	@ time	Ending Location	@ time	Route	Delays/ Detours
	Ending Odometer						
	Total Mileage						

reimbursement rate ¢/mile	fuel price $	costs to operate vehicle	tolls/fees	total hours	route notes
reimbursement total for today $	miles/gallon				

Pay Period: **Pay Date:**

Date	Starting Odometer	Starting Location	@ time	Ending Location	@ time	Route	Delays/Detours
	Ending Odometer						
	Total Mileage						

reimbursement rate ¢/mile	fuel price $	costs to operate vehicle	tolls/fees	total hours	route notes
reimbursement total for today $	miles/gallon				

Date	Starting Odometer	Starting Location	@ time	Ending Location	@ time	Route	Delays/Detours
	Ending Odometer						
	Total Mileage						

reimbursement rate ¢/mile	fuel price $	costs to operate vehicle	tolls/fees	total hours	route notes
reimbursement total for today $	miles/gallon				

Date	Starting Odometer	Starting Location	@ time	Ending Location	@ time	Route	Delays/Detours
	Ending Odometer						
	Total Mileage						

reimbursement rate ¢/mile	fuel price $	costs to operate vehicle	tolls/fees	total hours	route notes
reimbursement total for today $	miles/gallon				

Pay Period: **Pay Date:**

Entry 1

Date	Starting Odometer	Starting Location	@ time	Ending Location	@ time	Route	Delays/Detours
	Ending Odometer						
	Total Mileage						

reimbursement rate ¢/mile	fuel price $	costs to operate vehicle	tolls/fees	total hours	route notes
reimbursement total for today $	miles/gallon				

Entry 2

Date	Starting Odometer	Starting Location	@ time	Ending Location	@ time	Route	Delays/Detours
	Ending Odometer						
	Total Mileage						

reimbursement rate ¢/mile	fuel price $	costs to operate vehicle	tolls/fees	total hours	route notes
reimbursement total for today $	miles/gallon				

Entry 3

Date	Starting Odometer	Starting Location	@ time	Ending Location	@ time	Route	Delays/Detours
	Ending Odometer						
	Total Mileage						

reimbursement rate ¢/mile	fuel price $	costs to operate vehicle	tolls/fees	total hours	route notes
reimbursement total for today $	miles/gallon				

Pay Period: **Pay Date:**

Date	Starting Odometer	Starting Location	@ time	Ending Location	@ time	Route	Delays/Detours
	Ending Odometer						
	Total Mileage						

reimbursement rate ¢/mile	fuel price $	costs to operate vehicle	tolls/fees	total hours	route notes
reimbursement total for today $	miles/gallon				

Date	Starting Odometer	Starting Location	@ time	Ending Location	@ time	Route	Delays/Detours
	Ending Odometer						
	Total Mileage						

reimbursement rate ¢/mile	fuel price $	costs to operate vehicle	tolls/fees	total hours	route notes
reimbursement total for today $	miles/gallon				

Date	Starting Odometer	Starting Location	@ time	Ending Location	@ time	Route	Delays/Detours
	Ending Odometer						
	Total Mileage						

reimbursement rate ¢/mile	fuel price $	costs to operate vehicle	tolls/fees	total hours	route notes
reimbursement total for today $	miles/gallon				

this pay period

date range _____   pay date _____

date worked	hours worked	hourly rate	× tax rate (= net)	+ mileage	= total net

totals

total miles driven _____
total fuel costs $
total expenses $

Pay Period: **Pay Date:**

Date	Starting Odometer	Starting Location	@ time	Ending Location	@ time	Route	Delays/Detours
	Ending Odometer						
	Total Mileage						
reimbursement rate ¢/mile	fuel price $	costs to operate vehicle	tolls/fees	total hours	route notes		
reimbursement total for today $	miles/gallon						

Date	Starting Odometer	Starting Location	@ time	Ending Location	@ time	Route	Delays/Detours
	Ending Odometer						
	Total Mileage						
reimbursement rate ¢/mile	fuel price $	costs to operate vehicle	tolls/fees	total hours	route notes		
reimbursement total for today $	miles/gallon						

Date	Starting Odometer	Starting Location	@ time	Ending Location	@ time	Route	Delays/Detours
	Ending Odometer						
	Total Mileage						
reimbursement rate ¢/mile	fuel price $	costs to operate vehicle	tolls/fees	total hours	route notes		
reimbursement total for today $	miles/gallon						

Pay Period: **Pay Date:**

Date	Starting Odometer	Starting Location	@ time	Ending Location	@ time	Route	Delays/ Detours
	Ending Odometer						
	Total Mileage						

reimbursement rate ¢/mile	fuel price $	costs to operate vehicle	tolls/fees	total hours	route notes
reimbursement total for today $	miles/gallon				

Date	Starting Odometer	Starting Location	@ time	Ending Location	@ time	Route	Delays/ Detours
	Ending Odometer						
	Total Mileage						

reimbursement rate ¢/mile	fuel price $	costs to operate vehicle	tolls/fees	total hours	route notes
reimbursement total for today $	miles/gallon				

Date	Starting Odometer	Starting Location	@ time	Ending Location	@ time	Route	Delays/ Detours
	Ending Odometer						
	Total Mileage						

reimbursement rate ¢/mile	fuel price $	costs to operate vehicle	tolls/fees	total hours	route notes
reimbursement total for today $	miles/gallon				

Pay Period: **Pay Date:**

Date	Starting Odometer	Starting Location	@ time	Ending Location	@ time	Route	Delays/Detours
	Ending Odometer						
	Total Mileage						

reimbursement rate ¢/mile	fuel price $	costs to operate vehicle	tolls/fees	total hours	route notes
reimbursement total for today $	miles/gallon				

Date	Starting Odometer	Starting Location	@ time	Ending Location	@ time	Route	Delays/Detours
	Ending Odometer						
	Total Mileage						

reimbursement rate ¢/mile	fuel price $	costs to operate vehicle	tolls/fees	total hours	route notes
reimbursement total for today $	miles/gallon				

Date	Starting Odometer	Starting Location	@ time	Ending Location	@ time	Route	Delays/Detours
	Ending Odometer						
	Total Mileage						

reimbursement rate ¢/mile	fuel price $	costs to operate vehicle	tolls/fees	total hours	route notes
reimbursement total for today $	miles/gallon				

Pay Period: **Pay Date:**

Date	Starting Odometer	Starting Location	@ time	Ending Location	@ time	Route	Delays/Detours
	Ending Odometer						
	Total Mileage						
	reimbursement rate ¢/mile	fuel price $	costs to operate vehicle	tolls/fees	total hours	route notes	
	reimbursement total for today $	miles/gallon					

Date	Starting Odometer	Starting Location	@ time	Ending Location	@ time	Route	Delays/Detours
	Ending Odometer						
	Total Mileage						
	reimbursement rate ¢/mile	fuel price $	costs to operate vehicle	tolls/fees	total hours	route notes	
	reimbursement total for today $	miles/gallon					

Date	Starting Odometer	Starting Location	@ time	Ending Location	@ time	Route	Delays/Detours
	Ending Odometer						
	Total Mileage						
	reimbursement rate ¢/mile	fuel price $	costs to operate vehicle	tolls/fees	total hours	route notes	
	reimbursement total for today $	miles/gallon					

this pay period

date range _____   pay date _____

date worked	hours worked	hourly rate	× tax rate (= net)	+ mileage	= total net

totals

total miles driven _____
total fuel costs $
total expenses $

Pay Period: **Pay Date:**

Date	Starting Odometer	Starting Location	@ time	Ending Location	@ time	Route	Delays/Detours
	Ending Odometer					
	Total Mileage					

reimbursement rate ¢/mile	fuel price $	costs to operate vehicle	tolls/fees	total hours	route notes
reimbursement total for today $	miles/gallon				

Date	Starting Odometer	Starting Location	@ time	Ending Location	@ time	Route	Delays/Detours
	Ending Odometer					
	Total Mileage					

reimbursement rate ¢/mile	fuel price $	costs to operate vehicle	tolls/fees	total hours	route notes
reimbursement total for today $	miles/gallon				

Date	Starting Odometer	Starting Location	@ time	Ending Location	@ time	Route	Delays/Detours
	Ending Odometer					
	Total Mileage					

reimbursement rate ¢/mile	fuel price $	costs to operate vehicle	tolls/fees	total hours	route notes
reimbursement total for today $	miles/gallon				

Pay Period: **Pay Date:**

Date	Starting Odometer	Starting Location	@ time	Ending Location	@ time	Route	Delays/Detours
	Ending Odometer						
	Total Mileage						

reimbursement rate ¢/mile	fuel price $	costs to operate vehicle	tolls/fees	total hours	route notes
reimbursement total for today $	miles/gallon				

Date	Starting Odometer	Starting Location	@ time	Ending Location	@ time	Route	Delays/Detours
	Ending Odometer						
	Total Mileage						

reimbursement rate ¢/mile	fuel price $	costs to operate vehicle	tolls/fees	total hours	route notes
reimbursement total for today $	miles/gallon				

Date	Starting Odometer	Starting Location	@ time	Ending Location	@ time	Route	Delays/Detours
	Ending Odometer						
	Total Mileage						

reimbursement rate ¢/mile	fuel price $	costs to operate vehicle	tolls/fees	total hours	route notes
reimbursement total for today $	miles/gallon				

Pay Period: **Pay Date:**

Date	Starting Odometer	Starting Location	@ time	Ending Location	@ time	Route	Delays/Detours
	Ending Odometer						
	Total Mileage						
	reimbursement rate ¢/mile	fuel price $	costs to operate vehicle	tolls/fees	total hours	route notes	
	reimbursement total for today $	miles/gallon					

Date	Starting Odometer	Starting Location	@ time	Ending Location	@ time	Route	Delays/Detours
	Ending Odometer						
	Total Mileage						
	reimbursement rate ¢/mile	fuel price $	costs to operate vehicle	tolls/fees	total hours	route notes	
	reimbursement total for today $	miles/gallon					

Date	Starting Odometer	Starting Location	@ time	Ending Location	@ time	Route	Delays/Detours
	Ending Odometer						
	Total Mileage						
	reimbursement rate ¢/mile	fuel price $	costs to operate vehicle	tolls/fees	total hours	route notes	
	reimbursement total for today $	miles/gallon					

Pay Period: **Pay Date:**

Date	Starting Odometer	Starting Location	@ time	Ending Location	@ time	Route	Delays/Detours
	Ending Odometer						
	Total Mileage						

reimbursement rate ¢/mile	fuel price $	costs to operate vehicle	tolls/fees	total hours	route notes
reimbursement total for today $	miles/gallon				

Date	Starting Odometer	Starting Location	@ time	Ending Location	@ time	Route	Delays/Detours
	Ending Odometer						
	Total Mileage						

reimbursement rate ¢/mile	fuel price $	costs to operate vehicle	tolls/fees	total hours	route notes
reimbursement total for today $	miles/gallon				

Date	Starting Odometer	Starting Location	@ time	Ending Location	@ time	Route	Delays/Detours
	Ending Odometer						
	Total Mileage						

reimbursement rate ¢/mile	fuel price $	costs to operate vehicle	tolls/fees	total hours	route notes
reimbursement total for today $	miles/gallon				

this pay period

date range _____   pay date _____

date worked	hours worked	hourly rate	× tax rate (= net)	+ mileage	= total net

totals

total miles driven _____
total fuel costs $
total expenses $

Pay Period: **Pay Date:**

Date	Starting Odometer	Starting Location	@ time	Ending Location	@ time	Route	Delays/Detours
	Ending Odometer						
	Total Mileage						

reimbursement rate ¢/mile	fuel price $	costs to operate vehicle	tolls/fees	total hours	route notes
reimbursement total for today $	miles/gallon				

Date	Starting Odometer	Starting Location	@ time	Ending Location	@ time	Route	Delays/Detours
	Ending Odometer						
	Total Mileage						

reimbursement rate ¢/mile	fuel price $	costs to operate vehicle	tolls/fees	total hours	route notes
reimbursement total for today $	miles/gallon				

Date	Starting Odometer	Starting Location	@ time	Ending Location	@ time	Route	Delays/Detours
	Ending Odometer						
	Total Mileage						

reimbursement rate ¢/mile	fuel price $	costs to operate vehicle	tolls/fees	total hours	route notes
reimbursement total for today $	miles/gallon				

Pay Period: **Pay Date:**

Date	Starting Odometer	Starting Location	@ time	Ending Location	@ time	Route	Delays/ Detours
	Ending Odometer						
	Total Mileage						
	reimbursement rate ¢/mile	fuel price $	costs to operate vehicle	tolls/fees	total hours	route notes	
	reimbursement total for today $	miles/gallon					

Date	Starting Odometer	Starting Location	@ time	Ending Location	@ time	Route	Delays/ Detours
	Ending Odometer						
	Total Mileage						
	reimbursement rate ¢/mile	fuel price $	costs to operate vehicle	tolls/fees	total hours	route notes	
	reimbursement total for today $	miles/gallon					

Date	Starting Odometer	Starting Location	@ time	Ending Location	@ time	Route	Delays/ Detours
	Ending Odometer						
	Total Mileage						
	reimbursement rate ¢/mile	fuel price $	costs to operate vehicle	tolls/fees	total hours	route notes	
	reimbursement total for today $	miles/gallon					

Pay Period: **Pay Date:**

Date	Starting Odometer	Starting Location	@ time	Ending Location	@ time	Route	Delays/Detours
	Ending Odometer						
	Total Mileage						

reimbursement rate ¢/mile	fuel price $	costs to operate vehicle	tolls/fees	total hours	route notes
reimbursement total for today $	miles/gallon				

Date	Starting Odometer	Starting Location	@ time	Ending Location	@ time	Route	Delays/Detours
	Ending Odometer						
	Total Mileage						

reimbursement rate ¢/mile	fuel price $	costs to operate vehicle	tolls/fees	total hours	route notes
reimbursement total for today $	miles/gallon				

Date	Starting Odometer	Starting Location	@ time	Ending Location	@ time	Route	Delays/Detours
	Ending Odometer						
	Total Mileage						

reimbursement rate ¢/mile	fuel price $	costs to operate vehicle	tolls/fees	total hours	route notes
reimbursement total for today $	miles/gallon				

Pay Period: **Pay Date:**

Date	Starting Odometer	Starting Location	@ time	Ending Location	@ time	Route	Delays/ Detours
	Ending Odometer						
	Total Mileage						

reimbursement rate ¢/mile	fuel price $	costs to operate vehicle	tolls/fees	total hours	route notes
reimbursement total for today $	miles/gallon				

Date	Starting Odometer	Starting Location	@ time	Ending Location	@ time	Route	Delays/ Detours
	Ending Odometer						
	Total Mileage						

reimbursement rate ¢/mile	fuel price $	costs to operate vehicle	tolls/fees	total hours	route notes
reimbursement total for today $	miles/gallon				

Date	Starting Odometer	Starting Location	@ time	Ending Location	@ time	Route	Delays/ Detours
	Ending Odometer						
	Total Mileage						

reimbursement rate ¢/mile	fuel price $	costs to operate vehicle	tolls/fees	total hours	route notes
reimbursement total for today $	miles/gallon				

this pay period

date range _____   pay date _____

date worked	hours worked	hourly rate	× tax rate (= net)	+ mileage	= total net

totals

total miles driven _____
total fuel costs $
total expenses $

Pay Period: **Pay Date:**

Date	Starting Odometer	Starting Location	@ time	Ending Location	@ time	Route	Delays/Detours
	Ending Odometer						
	Total Mileage						
	reimbursement rate ¢/mile	fuel price $	costs to operate vehicle	tolls/fees	total hours	route notes	
	reimbursement total for today $	miles/gallon					

Date	Starting Odometer	Starting Location	@ time	Ending Location	@ time	Route	Delays/Detours
	Ending Odometer						
	Total Mileage						
	reimbursement rate ¢/mile	fuel price $	costs to operate vehicle	tolls/fees	total hours	route notes	
	reimbursement total for today $	miles/gallon					

Date	Starting Odometer	Starting Location	@ time	Ending Location	@ time	Route	Delays/Detours
	Ending Odometer						
	Total Mileage						
	reimbursement rate ¢/mile	fuel price $	costs to operate vehicle	tolls/fees	total hours	route notes	
	reimbursement total for today $	miles/gallon					

Pay Period: **Pay Date:**

Date	Starting Odometer	Starting Location	@ time	Ending Location	@ time	Route	Delays/ Detours
	Ending Odometer						
	Total Mileage						
	reimbursement rate ¢/mile	fuel price $	costs to operate vehicle	tolls/fees	total hours	route notes	
	reimbursement total for today $	miles/gallon					

Date	Starting Odometer	Starting Location	@ time	Ending Location	@ time	Route	Delays/ Detours
	Ending Odometer						
	Total Mileage						
	reimbursement rate ¢/mile	fuel price $	costs to operate vehicle	tolls/fees	total hours	route notes	
	reimbursement total for today $	miles/gallon					

Date	Starting Odometer	Starting Location	@ time	Ending Location	@ time	Route	Delays/ Detours
	Ending Odometer						
	Total Mileage						
	reimbursement rate ¢/mile	fuel price $	costs to operate vehicle	tolls/fees	total hours	route notes	
	reimbursement total for today $	miles/gallon					

Pay Period: **Pay Date:**

Date	Starting Odometer / Ending Odometer / Total Mileage	Starting Location	@ time	Ending Location	@ time	Route	Delays/ Detours
○							

reimbursement rate ¢/mile	fuel price $	costs to operate vehicle	tolls/fees	total hours	route notes
reimbursement total for today $	miles/gallon				

Date	Starting Odometer / Ending Odometer / Total Mileage	Starting Location	@ time	Ending Location	@ time	Route	Delays/ Detours
○							

reimbursement rate ¢/mile	fuel price $	costs to operate vehicle	tolls/fees	total hours	route notes
reimbursement total for today $	miles/gallon				

Date	Starting Odometer / Ending Odometer / Total Mileage	Starting Location	@ time	Ending Location	@ time	Route	Delays/ Detours
○							

reimbursement rate ¢/mile	fuel price $	costs to operate vehicle	tolls/fees	total hours	route notes
reimbursement total for today $	miles/gallon				

Pay Period: **Pay Date:**

Date	Starting Odometer	Starting Location	@ time	Ending Location	@ time	Route	Delays/ Detours
	Ending Odometer						
	Total Mileage						

reimbursement rate	fuel price	costs to operate vehicle	tolls/fees	total hours	route notes
¢/mile	$				
reimbursement total for today $	miles/gallon				

Date	Starting Odometer	Starting Location	@ time	Ending Location	@ time	Route	Delays/ Detours
	Ending Odometer						
	Total Mileage						

reimbursement rate	fuel price	costs to operate vehicle	tolls/fees	total hours	route notes
¢/mile	$				
reimbursement total for today $	miles/gallon				

Date	Starting Odometer	Starting Location	@ time	Ending Location	@ time	Route	Delays/ Detours
	Ending Odometer						
	Total Mileage						

reimbursement rate	fuel price	costs to operate vehicle	tolls/fees	total hours	route notes
¢/mile	$				
reimbursement total for today $	miles/gallon				

this pay period

date range _____   pay date _____

date worked	hours worked	hourly rate	× tax rate (= net)	+ mileage	= total net

totals

total miles driven _____
total fuel costs $
total expenses $

Pay Period: **Pay Date:**

Date	Starting Odometer	Starting Location	@ time	Ending Location	@ time	Route	Delays/Detours
	Ending Odometer						
	Total Mileage						

reimbursement rate ¢/mile	fuel price $	costs to operate vehicle	tolls/fees	total hours	route notes
reimbursement total for today $	miles/gallon				

Date	Starting Odometer	Starting Location	@ time	Ending Location	@ time	Route	Delays/Detours
	Ending Odometer						
	Total Mileage						

reimbursement rate ¢/mile	fuel price $	costs to operate vehicle	tolls/fees	total hours	route notes
reimbursement total for today $	miles/gallon				

Date	Starting Odometer	Starting Location	@ time	Ending Location	@ time	Route	Delays/Detours
	Ending Odometer						
	Total Mileage						

reimbursement rate ¢/mile	fuel price $	costs to operate vehicle	tolls/fees	total hours	route notes
reimbursement total for today $	miles/gallon				

Pay Period: **Pay Date:**

Date	Starting Odometer / Ending Odometer / Total Mileage	Starting Location	@ time	Ending Location	@ time	Route	Delays/ Detours
( )							

reimbursement rate ¢/mile
reimbursement total for today $

fuel price $
miles/gallon

costs to operate vehicle

tolls/fees

total hours

route notes

Date	Starting Odometer / Ending Odometer / Total Mileage	Starting Location	@ time	Ending Location	@ time	Route	Delays/ Detours
( )							

reimbursement rate ¢/mile
reimbursement total for today $

fuel price $
miles/gallon

costs to operate vehicle

tolls/fees

total hours

route notes

Date	Starting Odometer / Ending Odometer / Total Mileage	Starting Location	@ time	Ending Location	@ time	Route	Delays/ Detours
( )							

reimbursement rate ¢/mile
reimbursement total for today $

fuel price $
miles/gallon

costs to operate vehicle

tolls/fees

total hours

route notes

Pay Period: **Pay Date:**

Date	Starting Odometer	Starting Location	@ time	Ending Location	@ time	Route	Delays/Detours
	Ending Odometer						
	Total Mileage						

reimbursement rate ¢/mile	fuel price $	costs to operate vehicle	tolls/fees	total hours	route notes
reimbursement total for today $	miles/gallon				

Date	Starting Odometer	Starting Location	@ time	Ending Location	@ time	Route	Delays/Detours
	Ending Odometer						
	Total Mileage						

reimbursement rate ¢/mile	fuel price $	costs to operate vehicle	tolls/fees	total hours	route notes
reimbursement total for today $	miles/gallon				

Date	Starting Odometer	Starting Location	@ time	Ending Location	@ time	Route	Delays/Detours
	Ending Odometer						
	Total Mileage						

reimbursement rate ¢/mile	fuel price $	costs to operate vehicle	tolls/fees	total hours	route notes
reimbursement total for today $	miles/gallon				

Pay Period: **Pay Date:**

Date	Starting Odometer	Starting Location	@ time	Ending Location	@ time	Route	Delays/ Detours
○	Ending Odometer						
	Total Mileage						

reimbursement rate ¢/mile	fuel price $	costs to operate vehicle	tolls/fees	total hours	route notes
reimbursement total for today $	miles/gallon			□	

Date	Starting Odometer	Starting Location	@ time	Ending Location	@ time	Route	Delays/ Detours
○	Ending Odometer						
	Total Mileage						

reimbursement rate ¢/mile	fuel price $	costs to operate vehicle	tolls/fees	total hours	route notes
reimbursement total for today $	miles/gallon			□	

Date	Starting Odometer	Starting Location	@ time	Ending Location	@ time	Route	Delays/ Detours
○	Ending Odometer						
	Total Mileage						

reimbursement rate ¢/mile	fuel price $	costs to operate vehicle	tolls/fees	total hours	route notes
reimbursement total for today $	miles/gallon			□	

this pay period

date range _____   pay date _____

date worked	hours worked	hourly rate	× tax rate (= net)	+ mileage	= total net
totals					

total miles driven _____

total fuel costs $

total expenses $

Pay Period: **Pay Date:**

Date | Starting Odometer | Starting Location | @ time | Ending Location | @ time | Route | Delays/Detours

Ending Odometer

Total Mileage

reimbursement rate ¢/mile | fuel price $ | costs to operate vehicle | tolls/fees | total hours | route notes

reimbursement total for today $

Date | Starting Odometer | Starting Location | @ time | Ending Location | @ time | Route | Delays/Detours

Ending Odometer

Total Mileage

reimbursement rate ¢/mile | fuel price $ | costs to operate vehicle | tolls/fees | total hours | route notes

reimbursement total for today $

Date | Starting Odometer | Starting Location | @ time | Ending Location | @ time | Route | Delays/Detours

Ending Odometer

Total Mileage

reimbursement rate ¢/mile | fuel price $ | costs to operate vehicle | tolls/fees | total hours | route notes

reimbursement total for today $

Pay Period: **Pay Date:**

Entry 1

Date	Starting Odometer	Starting Location	@ time	Ending Location	@ time	Route	Delays/Detours
	Ending Odometer						
	Total Mileage						

reimbursement rate ¢/mile	fuel price $	costs to operate vehicle	tolls/fees	total hours	route notes
reimbursement total for today $	miles/gallon				

Entry 2

Date	Starting Odometer	Starting Location	@ time	Ending Location	@ time	Route	Delays/Detours
	Ending Odometer						
	Total Mileage						

reimbursement rate ¢/mile	fuel price $	costs to operate vehicle	tolls/fees	total hours	route notes
reimbursement total for today $	miles/gallon				

Entry 3

Date	Starting Odometer	Starting Location	@ time	Ending Location	@ time	Route	Delays/Detours
	Ending Odometer						
	Total Mileage						

reimbursement rate ¢/mile	fuel price $	costs to operate vehicle	tolls/fees	total hours	route notes
reimbursement total for today $	miles/gallon				

Pay Period: **Pay Date:**

Date	Starting Odometer	Starting Location	@ time	Ending Location	@ time	Route	Delays/ Detours
	Ending Odometer						
	Total Mileage						

reimbursement rate ¢/mile	fuel price $	costs to operate vehicle	tolls/fees	total hours	route notes
reimbursement total for today $	miles/gallon				

Date	Starting Odometer	Starting Location	@ time	Ending Location	@ time	Route	Delays/ Detours
	Ending Odometer						
	Total Mileage						

reimbursement rate ¢/mile	fuel price $	costs to operate vehicle	tolls/fees	total hours	route notes
reimbursement total for today $	miles/gallon				

Date	Starting Odometer	Starting Location	@ time	Ending Location	@ time	Route	Delays/ Detours
	Ending Odometer						
	Total Mileage						

reimbursement rate ¢/mile	fuel price $	costs to operate vehicle	tolls/fees	total hours	route notes
reimbursement total for today $	miles/gallon				

Pay Period: **Pay Date:**

Date	Starting Odometer	Starting Location	@ time	Ending Location	@ time	Route	Delays/ Detours
	Ending Odometer						
	Total Mileage						

reimbursement rate ¢/mile	fuel price $	costs to operate vehicle	tolls/fees	total hours	route notes
reimbursement total for today $	miles/gallon				

Date	Starting Odometer	Starting Location	@ time	Ending Location	@ time	Route	Delays/ Detours
	Ending Odometer						
	Total Mileage						

reimbursement rate ¢/mile	fuel price $	costs to operate vehicle	tolls/fees	total hours	route notes
reimbursement total for today $	miles/gallon				

Date	Starting Odometer	Starting Location	@ time	Ending Location	@ time	Route	Delays/ Detours
	Ending Odometer						
	Total Mileage						

reimbursement rate ¢/mile	fuel price $	costs to operate vehicle	tolls/fees	total hours	route notes
reimbursement total for today $	miles/gallon				

this pay period

date range _____   pay date _____

			×		
date worked	hours worked	hourly rate	tax rate (= net)	+ mileage	= total net
totals					

total miles driven _____

total fuel costs $

total expenses $

Pay Period: **Pay Date:**

Date	Starting Odometer	Starting Location	@ time	Ending Location	@ time	Route	Delays/Detours
	Ending Odometer						
	Total Mileage						

| reimbursement rate ¢/mile | fuel price $ | costs to operate vehicle | tolls/fees | total hours | route notes | | |
| reimbursement total for today $ | miles/gallon | | | | | | |

Date	Starting Odometer	Starting Location	@ time	Ending Location	@ time	Route	Delays/Detours
	Ending Odometer						
	Total Mileage						

| reimbursement rate ¢/mile | fuel price $ | costs to operate vehicle | tolls/fees | total hours | route notes | | |
| reimbursement total for today $ | miles/gallon | | | | | | |

Date	Starting Odometer	Starting Location	@ time	Ending Location	@ time	Route	Delays/Detours
	Ending Odometer						
	Total Mileage						

| reimbursement rate ¢/mile | fuel price $ | costs to operate vehicle | tolls/fees | total hours | route notes | | |
| reimbursement total for today $ | miles/gallon | | | | | | |

Pay Period:　　　　　　　　　　　　　　　**Pay Date:**

Date	Starting Odometer	Starting Location	@ time	Ending Location	@ time	Route	Delays/ Detours
	Ending Odometer						
	Total Mileage						

reimbursement rate ¢/mile	fuel price $	costs to operate vehicle	tolls/fees	total hours	route notes
reimbursement total for today $	miles/gallon				

Date	Starting Odometer	Starting Location	@ time	Ending Location	@ time	Route	Delays/ Detours
	Ending Odometer						
	Total Mileage						

reimbursement rate ¢/mile	fuel price $	costs to operate vehicle	tolls/fees	total hours	route notes
reimbursement total for today $	miles/gallon				

Date	Starting Odometer	Starting Location	@ time	Ending Location	@ time	Route	Delays/ Detours
	Ending Odometer						
	Total Mileage						

reimbursement rate ¢/mile	fuel price $	costs to operate vehicle	tolls/fees	total hours	route notes
reimbursement total for today $	miles/gallon				

Pay Period: **Pay Date:**

Entry 1

Date	Starting Odometer	Starting Location	@ time	Ending Location	@ time	Route	Delays/Detours
	Ending Odometer						
	Total Mileage						

- reimbursement rate: ¢/mile
- fuel price: $
- costs to operate vehicle
- tolls/fees
- total hours
- route notes
- reimbursement total for today: $
- miles/gallon

Entry 2

Date	Starting Odometer	Starting Location	@ time	Ending Location	@ time	Route	Delays/Detours
	Ending Odometer						
	Total Mileage						

- reimbursement rate: ¢/mile
- fuel price: $
- costs to operate vehicle
- tolls/fees
- total hours
- route notes
- reimbursement total for today: $
- miles/gallon

Entry 3

Date	Starting Odometer	Starting Location	@ time	Ending Location	@ time	Route	Delays/Detours
	Ending Odometer						
	Total Mileage						

- reimbursement rate: ¢/mile
- fuel price: $
- costs to operate vehicle
- tolls/fees
- total hours
- route notes
- reimbursement total for today: $
- miles/gallon

Pay Period: **Pay Date:**

Date	Starting Odometer	Starting Location	@ time	Ending Location	@ time	Route	Delays/ Detours
○	Ending Odometer						
	Total Mileage						

reimbursement rate ¢/mile	fuel price $	costs to operate vehicle	tolls/fees	total hours ☐	route notes		
reimbursement total for today $	miles/gallon						

Date	Starting Odometer	Starting Location	@ time	Ending Location	@ time	Route	Delays/ Detours
○	Ending Odometer						
	Total Mileage						

reimbursement rate ¢/mile	fuel price $	costs to operate vehicle	tolls/fees	total hours ☐	route notes		
reimbursement total for today $	miles/gallon						

Date	Starting Odometer	Starting Location	@ time	Ending Location	@ time	Route	Delays/ Detours
○	Ending Odometer						
	Total Mileage						

reimbursement rate ¢/mile	fuel price $	costs to operate vehicle	tolls/fees	total hours ☐	route notes		
reimbursement total for today $	miles/gallon						

this pay period

date range _____   pay date _____

date worked	hours worked	hourly rate	× tax rate (= net)	+ mileage	= total net

totals

total miles driven _____
total fuel costs $
total expenses $

Pay Period: **Pay Date:**

Date	Starting Odometer	Starting Location	@ time	Ending Location	@ time	Route	Delays/ Detours
	Ending Odometer						
	Total Mileage						

reimbursement rate ¢/mile	fuel price $	costs to operate vehicle	tolls/fees	total hours	route notes
reimbursement total for today $	miles/gallon				

Date	Starting Odometer	Starting Location	@ time	Ending Location	@ time	Route	Delays/ Detours
	Ending Odometer						
	Total Mileage						

reimbursement rate ¢/mile	fuel price $	costs to operate vehicle	tolls/fees	total hours	route notes
reimbursement total for today $	miles/gallon				

Date	Starting Odometer	Starting Location	@ time	Ending Location	@ time	Route	Delays/ Detours
	Ending Odometer						
	Total Mileage						

reimbursement rate ¢/mile	fuel price $	costs to operate vehicle	tolls/fees	total hours	route notes
reimbursement total for today $	miles/gallon				

Pay Period: **Pay Date:**

Date	Starting Odometer	Starting Location	@ time	Ending Location	@ time	Route	Delays/ Detours
	Ending Odometer						
	Total Mileage						

reimbursement rate ¢/mile	fuel price $	costs to operate vehicle	tolls/fees	total hours	route notes
reimbursement total for today $	miles/gallon				

Date	Starting Odometer	Starting Location	@ time	Ending Location	@ time	Route	Delays/ Detours
	Ending Odometer						
	Total Mileage						

reimbursement rate ¢/mile	fuel price $	costs to operate vehicle	tolls/fees	total hours	route notes
reimbursement total for today $	miles/gallon				

Date	Starting Odometer	Starting Location	@ time	Ending Location	@ time	Route	Delays/ Detours
	Ending Odometer						
	Total Mileage						

reimbursement rate ¢/mile	fuel price $	costs to operate vehicle	tolls/fees	total hours	route notes
reimbursement total for today $	miles/gallon				

Pay Period: **Pay Date:**

Date	Starting Odometer	Starting Location	@ time	Ending Location	@ time	Route	Delays/ Detours
	Ending Odometer						
	Total Mileage						

reimbursement rate ¢/mile	fuel price $	costs to operate vehicle	tolls/fees	total hours	route notes
reimbursement total for today $	miles/gallon				

Date	Starting Odometer	Starting Location	@ time	Ending Location	@ time	Route	Delays/ Detours
	Ending Odometer						
	Total Mileage						

reimbursement rate ¢/mile	fuel price $	costs to operate vehicle	tolls/fees	total hours	route notes
reimbursement total for today $	miles/gallon				

Date	Starting Odometer	Starting Location	@ time	Ending Location	@ time	Route	Delays/ Detours
	Ending Odometer						
	Total Mileage						

reimbursement rate ¢/mile	fuel price $	costs to operate vehicle	tolls/fees	total hours	route notes
reimbursement total for today $	miles/gallon				

Pay Period:　　　　　　　　　　　　　　　　　**Pay Date:**

Date	Starting Odometer	Starting Location	@ time	Ending Location	@ time	Route	Delays/ Detours
	Ending Odometer						
	Total Mileage						

reimbursement rate ¢/mile	fuel price $	costs to operate vehicle	tolls/fees	total hours	route notes
reimbursement total for today $	miles/gallon				

Date	Starting Odometer	Starting Location	@ time	Ending Location	@ time	Route	Delays/ Detours
	Ending Odometer						
	Total Mileage						

reimbursement rate ¢/mile	fuel price $	costs to operate vehicle	tolls/fees	total hours	route notes
reimbursement total for today $	miles/gallon				

Date	Starting Odometer	Starting Location	@ time	Ending Location	@ time	Route	Delays/ Detours
	Ending Odometer						
	Total Mileage						

reimbursement rate ¢/mile	fuel price $	costs to operate vehicle	tolls/fees	total hours	route notes
reimbursement total for today $	miles/gallon				

this pay period

date range _____   pay date _____

date worked	hours worked	hourly rate	× tax rate (= net)	+ mileage	= total net

totals

total miles driven _____

total fuel costs $

total expenses $

Pay Period: **Pay Date:**

Date	Starting Odometer	Starting Location	@ time	Ending Location	@ time	Route	Delays/Detours
	Ending Odometer						
	Total Mileage						

reimbursement rate ¢/mile	fuel price $	costs to operate vehicle	tolls/fees	total hours	route notes
reimbursement total for today $	miles/gallon				

Date	Starting Odometer	Starting Location	@ time	Ending Location	@ time	Route	Delays/Detours
	Ending Odometer						
	Total Mileage						

reimbursement rate ¢/mile	fuel price $	costs to operate vehicle	tolls/fees	total hours	route notes
reimbursement total for today $	miles/gallon				

Date	Starting Odometer	Starting Location	@ time	Ending Location	@ time	Route	Delays/Detours
	Ending Odometer						
	Total Mileage						

reimbursement rate ¢/mile	fuel price $	costs to operate vehicle	tolls/fees	total hours	route notes
reimbursement total for today $	miles/gallon				

Pay Period: **Pay Date:**

Date	Starting Odometer	Starting Location	@ time	Ending Location	@ time	Route	Delays/ Detours
	Ending Odometer						
	Total Mileage						

reimbursement rate ¢/mile	fuel price $	costs to operate vehicle	tolls/fees	total hours	route notes
reimbursement total for today $	miles/gallon				

Date	Starting Odometer	Starting Location	@ time	Ending Location	@ time	Route	Delays/ Detours
	Ending Odometer						
	Total Mileage						

reimbursement rate ¢/mile	fuel price $	costs to operate vehicle	tolls/fees	total hours	route notes
reimbursement total for today $	miles/gallon				

Date	Starting Odometer	Starting Location	@ time	Ending Location	@ time	Route	Delays/ Detours
	Ending Odometer						
	Total Mileage						

reimbursement rate ¢/mile	fuel price $	costs to operate vehicle	tolls/fees	total hours	route notes
reimbursement total for today $	miles/gallon				

Pay Period: **Pay Date:**

Date	Starting Odometer / Ending Odometer / Total Mileage	Starting Location	@ time	Ending Location	@ time	Route	Delays/ Detours
○							

reimbursement rate ¢/mile
reimbursement total for today $

fuel price $
miles/gallon

costs to operate vehicle

tolls/fees

total hours

route notes

Date	Starting Odometer / Ending Odometer / Total Mileage	Starting Location	@ time	Ending Location	@ time	Route	Delays/ Detours
○							

reimbursement rate ¢/mile
reimbursement total for today $

fuel price $
miles/gallon

costs to operate vehicle

tolls/fees

total hours

route notes

Date	Starting Odometer / Ending Odometer / Total Mileage	Starting Location	@ time	Ending Location	@ time	Route	Delays/ Detours
○							

reimbursement rate ¢/mile
reimbursement total for today $

fuel price $
miles/gallon

costs to operate vehicle

tolls/fees

total hours

route notes

Pay Period: **Pay Date:**

Entry 1

Date	Starting Odometer	Starting Location	@ time	Ending Location	@ time	Route	Delays/Detours
	Ending Odometer						
	Total Mileage						

reimbursement rate	fuel price	costs to operate vehicle	tolls/fees	total hours	route notes
¢/mile	$				
reimbursement total for today	miles/gallon				
$					

Entry 2

Date	Starting Odometer	Starting Location	@ time	Ending Location	@ time	Route	Delays/Detours
	Ending Odometer						
	Total Mileage						

reimbursement rate	fuel price	costs to operate vehicle	tolls/fees	total hours	route notes
¢/mile	$				
reimbursement total for today	miles/gallon				
$					

Entry 3

Date	Starting Odometer	Starting Location	@ time	Ending Location	@ time	Route	Delays/Detours
	Ending Odometer						
	Total Mileage						

reimbursement rate	fuel price	costs to operate vehicle	tolls/fees	total hours	route notes
¢/mile	$				
reimbursement total for today	miles/gallon				
$					

this pay period

date range _____   pay date _____

date worked	hours worked	hourly rate	× tax rate (= net)	+ mileage	= total net

totals

total miles driven _____
total fuel costs $
total expenses $

Pay Period: **Pay Date:**

Date	Starting Odometer	Starting Location	@ time	Ending Location	@ time	Route	Delays/Detours
	Ending Odometer						
	Total Mileage						

reimbursement rate ¢/mile	fuel price $	costs to operate vehicle	tolls/fees	total hours	route notes
reimbursement total for today $	miles/gallon				

Date	Starting Odometer	Starting Location	@ time	Ending Location	@ time	Route	Delays/Detours
	Ending Odometer						
	Total Mileage						

reimbursement rate ¢/mile	fuel price $	costs to operate vehicle	tolls/fees	total hours	route notes
reimbursement total for today $	miles/gallon				

Date	Starting Odometer	Starting Location	@ time	Ending Location	@ time	Route	Delays/Detours
	Ending Odometer						
	Total Mileage						

reimbursement rate ¢/mile	fuel price $	costs to operate vehicle	tolls/fees	total hours	route notes
reimbursement total for today $	miles/gallon				

Pay Period: **Pay Date:**

Date	Starting Odometer	Starting Location	@ time	Ending Location	@ time	Route	Delays/Detours
	Ending Odometer						
	Total Mileage						

reimbursement rate ¢/mile	fuel price $	costs to operate vehicle	tolls/fees	total hours	route notes
reimbursement total for today $	miles/gallon				

Date	Starting Odometer	Starting Location	@ time	Ending Location	@ time	Route	Delays/Detours
	Ending Odometer						
	Total Mileage						

reimbursement rate ¢/mile	fuel price $	costs to operate vehicle	tolls/fees	total hours	route notes
reimbursement total for today $	miles/gallon				

Date	Starting Odometer	Starting Location	@ time	Ending Location	@ time	Route	Delays/Detours
	Ending Odometer						
	Total Mileage						

reimbursement rate ¢/mile	fuel price $	costs to operate vehicle	tolls/fees	total hours	route notes
reimbursement total for today $	miles/gallon				

Pay Period:　　　　　　　　　　　　　　　　**Pay Date:**

Date	Starting Odometer	Starting Location	@ time	Ending Location	@ time	Route	Delays/ Detours
	Ending Odometer						
	Total Mileage						

reimbursement rate ¢/mile	fuel price $	costs to operate vehicle	tolls/fees	total hours	route notes
reimbursement total for today $	miles/gallon				

Date	Starting Odometer	Starting Location	@ time	Ending Location	@ time	Route	Delays/ Detours
	Ending Odometer						
	Total Mileage						

reimbursement rate ¢/mile	fuel price $	costs to operate vehicle	tolls/fees	total hours	route notes
reimbursement total for today $	miles/gallon				

Date	Starting Odometer	Starting Location	@ time	Ending Location	@ time	Route	Delays/ Detours
	Ending Odometer						
	Total Mileage						

reimbursement rate ¢/mile	fuel price $	costs to operate vehicle	tolls/fees	total hours	route notes
reimbursement total for today $	miles/gallon				

Pay Period: **Pay Date:**

Date	Starting Odometer	Starting Location	@ time	Ending Location	@ time	Route	Delays/Detours
	Ending Odometer					
	Total Mileage					

| reimbursement rate ¢/mile | fuel price $ | costs to operate vehicle | tolls/fees | total hours | route notes |
| reimbursement total for today $ | miles/gallon | | | | |

Date	Starting Odometer	Starting Location	@ time	Ending Location	@ time	Route	Delays/Detours
	Ending Odometer					
	Total Mileage					

| reimbursement rate ¢/mile | fuel price $ | costs to operate vehicle | tolls/fees | total hours | route notes |
| reimbursement total for today $ | miles/gallon | | | | |

Date	Starting Odometer	Starting Location	@ time	Ending Location	@ time	Route	Delays/Detours
	Ending Odometer					
	Total Mileage					

| reimbursement rate ¢/mile | fuel price $ | costs to operate vehicle | tolls/fees | total hours | route notes |
| reimbursement total for today $ | miles/gallon | | | | |

this pay period

date range _____   pay date _____

date worked	hours worked	hourly rate	× tax rate (= net)	+ mileage	= total net

totals

total miles driven _____
total fuel costs $
total expenses $

Pay Period: **Pay Date:**

Date	Starting Odometer	Starting Location	@ time	Ending Location	@ time	Route	Delays/Detours
	Ending Odometer						
	Total Mileage						
reimbursement rate ¢/mile	fuel price $	costs to operate vehicle	tolls/fees	total hours	route notes		
reimbursement total for today $	miles/gallon						

Date	Starting Odometer	Starting Location	@ time	Ending Location	@ time	Route	Delays/Detours
	Ending Odometer						
	Total Mileage						
reimbursement rate ¢/mile	fuel price $	costs to operate vehicle	tolls/fees	total hours	route notes		
reimbursement total for today $	miles/gallon						

Date	Starting Odometer	Starting Location	@ time	Ending Location	@ time	Route	Delays/Detours
	Ending Odometer						
	Total Mileage						
reimbursement rate ¢/mile	fuel price $	costs to operate vehicle	tolls/fees	total hours	route notes		
reimbursement total for today $	miles/gallon						

Pay Period: **Pay Date:**

Date	Starting Odometer	Starting Location	@ time	Ending Location	@ time	Route	Delays/ Detours
	Ending Odometer						
	Total Mileage						
	reimbursement rate ¢/mile	fuel price $	costs to operate vehicle	tolls/fees	total hours	route notes	
	reimbursement total for today $	miles/gallon					

Date	Starting Odometer	Starting Location	@ time	Ending Location	@ time	Route	Delays/ Detours
	Ending Odometer						
	Total Mileage						
	reimbursement rate ¢/mile	fuel price $	costs to operate vehicle	tolls/fees	total hours	route notes	
	reimbursement total for today $	miles/gallon					

Date	Starting Odometer	Starting Location	@ time	Ending Location	@ time	Route	Delays/ Detours
	Ending Odometer						
	Total Mileage						
	reimbursement rate ¢/mile	fuel price $	costs to operate vehicle	tolls/fees	total hours	route notes	
	reimbursement total for today $	miles/gallon					

Pay Period: **Pay Date:**

Date	Starting Odometer	Starting Location	@ time	Ending Location	@ time	Route	Delays/Detours
	Ending Odometer						
	Total Mileage						

reimbursement rate ¢/mile	fuel price $	costs to operate vehicle	tolls/fees	total hours	route notes
reimbursement total for today $	miles/gallon				

Date	Starting Odometer	Starting Location	@ time	Ending Location	@ time	Route	Delays/Detours
	Ending Odometer						
	Total Mileage						

reimbursement rate ¢/mile	fuel price $	costs to operate vehicle	tolls/fees	total hours	route notes
reimbursement total for today $	miles/gallon				

Date	Starting Odometer	Starting Location	@ time	Ending Location	@ time	Route	Delays/Detours
	Ending Odometer						
	Total Mileage						

reimbursement rate ¢/mile	fuel price $	costs to operate vehicle	tolls/fees	total hours	route notes
reimbursement total for today $	miles/gallon				

Pay Period: **Pay Date:**

Date	Starting Odometer	Starting Location	@ time	Ending Location	@ time	Route	Delays/ Detours
	Ending Odometer						
	Total Mileage						

reimbursement rate ¢/mile	fuel price $	costs to operate vehicle	tolls/fees	total hours	route notes
reimbursement total for today $	miles/gallon				

Date	Starting Odometer	Starting Location	@ time	Ending Location	@ time	Route	Delays/ Detours
	Ending Odometer						
	Total Mileage						

reimbursement rate ¢/mile	fuel price $	costs to operate vehicle	tolls/fees	total hours	route notes
reimbursement total for today $	miles/gallon				

Date	Starting Odometer	Starting Location	@ time	Ending Location	@ time	Route	Delays/ Detours
	Ending Odometer						
	Total Mileage						

reimbursement rate ¢/mile	fuel price $	costs to operate vehicle	tolls/fees	total hours	route notes
reimbursement total for today $	miles/gallon				

this pay period

date range _____   pay date _____

date worked	hours worked	hourly rate	x tax rate (= net)	+ mileage	= total net

totals

total miles driven _____

total fuel costs $

total expenses $

Pay Period: **Pay Date:**

Date	Starting Odometer	Starting Location	@ time	Ending Location	@ time	Route	Delays/Detours
	Ending Odometer					
	Total Mileage					

reimbursement rate ¢/mile	fuel price $	costs to operate vehicle	tolls/fees	total hours	route notes
reimbursement total for today $	miles/gallon				

Date	Starting Odometer	Starting Location	@ time	Ending Location	@ time	Route	Delays/Detours
	Ending Odometer					
	Total Mileage					

reimbursement rate ¢/mile	fuel price $	costs to operate vehicle	tolls/fees	total hours	route notes
reimbursement total for today $	miles/gallon				

Date	Starting Odometer	Starting Location	@ time	Ending Location	@ time	Route	Delays/Detours
	Ending Odometer					
	Total Mileage					

reimbursement rate ¢/mile	fuel price $	costs to operate vehicle	tolls/fees	total hours	route notes
reimbursement total for today $	miles/gallon				

Pay Period: **Pay Date:**

Date	Starting Odometer	Starting Location	@ time	Ending Location	@ time	Route	Delays/ Detours
	Ending Odometer						
	Total Mileage						
reimbursement rate ¢/mile	fuel price $	costs to operate vehicle	tolls/fees	total hours	route notes		
reimbursement total for today $	miles/gallon						

Date	Starting Odometer	Starting Location	@ time	Ending Location	@ time	Route	Delays/ Detours
	Ending Odometer						
	Total Mileage						
reimbursement rate ¢/mile	fuel price $	costs to operate vehicle	tolls/fees	total hours	route notes		
reimbursement total for today $	miles/gallon						

Date	Starting Odometer	Starting Location	@ time	Ending Location	@ time	Route	Delays/ Detours
	Ending Odometer						
	Total Mileage						
reimbursement rate ¢/mile	fuel price $	costs to operate vehicle	tolls/fees	total hours	route notes		
reimbursement total for today $	miles/gallon						

Pay Period: **Pay Date:**

Date	Starting Odometer	Starting Location	@ time	Ending Location	@ time	Route	Delays/Detours
	Ending Odometer						
	Total Mileage						

reimbursement rate ¢/mile	fuel price $	costs to operate vehicle	tolls/fees	total hours	route notes
reimbursement total for today $	miles/gallon				

Date	Starting Odometer	Starting Location	@ time	Ending Location	@ time	Route	Delays/Detours
	Ending Odometer						
	Total Mileage						

reimbursement rate ¢/mile	fuel price $	costs to operate vehicle	tolls/fees	total hours	route notes
reimbursement total for today $	miles/gallon				

Date	Starting Odometer	Starting Location	@ time	Ending Location	@ time	Route	Delays/Detours
	Ending Odometer						
	Total Mileage						

reimbursement rate ¢/mile	fuel price $	costs to operate vehicle	tolls/fees	total hours	route notes
reimbursement total for today $	miles/gallon				

Pay Period: **Pay Date:**

Date	Starting Odometer	Starting Location	@ time	Ending Location	@ time	Route	Delays/Detours
	Ending Odometer						
	Total Mileage						

reimbursement rate ¢/mile	fuel price $	costs to operate vehicle	tolls/fees	total hours	route notes
reimbursement total for today $	miles/gallon				

Date	Starting Odometer	Starting Location	@ time	Ending Location	@ time	Route	Delays/Detours
	Ending Odometer						
	Total Mileage						

reimbursement rate ¢/mile	fuel price $	costs to operate vehicle	tolls/fees	total hours	route notes
reimbursement total for today $	miles/gallon				

Date	Starting Odometer	Starting Location	@ time	Ending Location	@ time	Route	Delays/Detours
	Ending Odometer						
	Total Mileage						

reimbursement rate ¢/mile	fuel price $	costs to operate vehicle	tolls/fees	total hours	route notes
reimbursement total for today $	miles/gallon				

this pay period

date range _____   pay date _____

date worked	hours worked	hourly rate	× tax rate (= net)	+ mileage	= total net
totals					

total miles driven _____
total fuel costs $
total expenses $

Pay Period: **Pay Date:**

Entry 1

Date	Starting Odometer	Starting Location	@ time	Ending Location	@ time	Route	Delays/Detours
	Ending Odometer						
	Total Mileage						

reimbursement rate ¢/mile	fuel price $	costs to operate vehicle	tolls/fees	total hours	route notes
reimbursement total for today $	miles/gallon				

Entry 2

Date	Starting Odometer	Starting Location	@ time	Ending Location	@ time	Route	Delays/Detours
	Ending Odometer						
	Total Mileage						

reimbursement rate ¢/mile	fuel price $	costs to operate vehicle	tolls/fees	total hours	route notes
reimbursement total for today $	miles/gallon				

Entry 3

Date	Starting Odometer	Starting Location	@ time	Ending Location	@ time	Route	Delays/Detours
	Ending Odometer						
	Total Mileage						

reimbursement rate ¢/mile	fuel price $	costs to operate vehicle	tolls/fees	total hours	route notes
reimbursement total for today $	miles/gallon				

Pay Period: **Pay Date:**

Date	Starting Odometer / Ending Odometer / Total Mileage	Starting Location	@ time	Ending Location	@ time	Route	Delays/ Detours

reimbursement rate ¢/mile	fuel price $	costs to operate vehicle	tolls/fees	total hours	route notes
reimbursement total for today $	miles/gallon				

Date	Starting Odometer / Ending Odometer / Total Mileage	Starting Location	@ time	Ending Location	@ time	Route	Delays/ Detours

reimbursement rate ¢/mile	fuel price $	costs to operate vehicle	tolls/fees	total hours	route notes
reimbursement total for today $	miles/gallon				

Date	Starting Odometer / Ending Odometer / Total Mileage	Starting Location	@ time	Ending Location	@ time	Route	Delays/ Detours

reimbursement rate ¢/mile	fuel price $	costs to operate vehicle	tolls/fees	total hours	route notes
reimbursement total for today $	miles/gallon				

Pay Period: **Pay Date:**

Date	Starting Odometer	Starting Location	@ time	Ending Location	@ time	Route	Delays/Detours
	Ending Odometer						
	Total Mileage						
	reimbursement rate ¢/mile	fuel price $	costs to operate vehicle	tolls/fees	total hours	route notes	
	reimbursement total for today $	miles/gallon					

Date	Starting Odometer	Starting Location	@ time	Ending Location	@ time	Route	Delays/Detours
	Ending Odometer						
	Total Mileage						
	reimbursement rate ¢/mile	fuel price $	costs to operate vehicle	tolls/fees	total hours	route notes	
	reimbursement total for today $	miles/gallon					

Date	Starting Odometer	Starting Location	@ time	Ending Location	@ time	Route	Delays/Detours
	Ending Odometer						
	Total Mileage						
	reimbursement rate ¢/mile	fuel price $	costs to operate vehicle	tolls/fees	total hours	route notes	
	reimbursement total for today $	miles/gallon					

Pay Period: **Pay Date:**

Date	Starting Odometer	Starting Location	@ time	Ending Location	@ time	Route	Delays/Detours
	Ending Odometer						
	Total Mileage						

reimbursement rate ¢/mile	fuel price $	costs to operate vehicle	tolls/fees	total hours	route notes
reimbursement total for today $	miles/gallon				

Date	Starting Odometer	Starting Location	@ time	Ending Location	@ time	Route	Delays/Detours
	Ending Odometer						
	Total Mileage						

reimbursement rate ¢/mile	fuel price $	costs to operate vehicle	tolls/fees	total hours	route notes
reimbursement total for today $	miles/gallon				

Date	Starting Odometer	Starting Location	@ time	Ending Location	@ time	Route	Delays/Detours
	Ending Odometer						
	Total Mileage						

reimbursement rate ¢/mile	fuel price $	costs to operate vehicle	tolls/fees	total hours	route notes
reimbursement total for today $	miles/gallon				

this pay period

date range _____ pay date _____

date worked	hours worked	hourly rate	× tax rate (= net)	+ mileage	= total net

totals

total miles driven _____

total fuel costs $

total expenses $

www.ingramcontent.com/pod-product-compliance
Lightning Source LLC
Chambersburg PA
CBHW080550220526
45466CB00010B/3098